Breathe Well
and Live Well
with COPD

of related interest

Chair Yoga
Seated Exercises for Health and Wellbeing
Edeltraud Rohnfeld
ISBN 978 1 84819 078 8
eISBN 978 0 85701 056 8

How to Give Clients the Skills to Stop Panic Attacks
Don't Forget to Breathe
Sandra Scheinbaum
ISBN 978 1 84905 887 2
eISBN 978 0 85700 603 5

Principles of the Alexander Technique
What it is, how it works, and what it can do for you
2nd edition
Jeremy Chance
Foreword by Dr David Garlick
ISBN 978 1 84819 128 0
eISBN 978 0 85701 105 3

Seated Taiji and Qigong
Guided Therapeutic Exercises to Manage Stress
and Balance Mind, Body and Spirit
Cynthia W. Quarta
Foreword by Michelle Maloney Vallie
ISBN 978 1 84819 088 7
eISBN 978 0 85701 071 1

Breathe Well and Live Well with COPD

A 28-Day Breathing Exercise Plan

Janet Brindley

Foreword by Linda Shampan

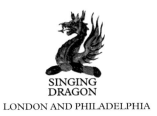

SINGING
DRAGON

LONDON AND PHILADELPHIA

First published in 2014
by Singing Dragon
an imprint of Jessica Kingsley Publishers
116 Pentonville Road
London N1 9JB, UK
and
400 Market Street, Suite 400
Philadelphia, PA 19106, USA

www.singingdragon.com

Library of Congress Cataloging in Publication Data
A CIP catalog record for this book is available from the Library of Congress

British Library Cataloguing in Publication Data
A CIP catalogue record for this book is available from the British Library

ISBN 978 1 84819 164 8
eISBN 978 0 85701 132 9

Printed and bound in China

Contents

Foreword
A personal experience of using breathing techniques

In my younger days I'd trained as a nurse, so I thought I already understood the basics of lungs and breathing. What a life-changing surprise it was, many years later at the age of 50, to find a breathing teacher who showed me the essentials of how to really breathe efficiently and to improve my quality of life; I had long-standing asthma and a recent diagnosis of moderate Chronic Obstructive Pulmonary Disease (COPD).

The three key breathing elements which transformed my health were changing to nose-breathing, learning how to keep breaths gentle and controlled, and breathing into my lower chest. All of these are covered in this book.

Now, aged 63, I appreciate that having the benefit of these breathing exercises has enabled me to live well with COPD, to continue working, to engage in physical activities such as yoga, and to enjoy a varied social life.

Breathing and emotions are closely connected, and feeling short of breath can trigger a range of feelings, such as anxiety, fear or frustration; for me the hardest one is feeling irritable. I find it helps to acknowledge to myself whatever the feeling is, give it time to settle and sometimes I explain to other people that I just need some time, on my own, to sort the breathing out.

I am lucky to have a supportive doctor who has shown interest and encouraged me in these self-help methods, alongside using conventional medication on an ongoing basis. What else helped me? Singing – in groups and workshops!

Linda Shampan
UKCP Registered Psychotherapist
and qualified Buteyko teacher

Acknowledgements

My first debt is to all the people who have been in my breathing classes: patients, students, teachers and men, women and children with breathing problems who have helped me to modify my teaching to meet their needs.

I am particularly grateful to Kathryn Godfrey, Dr James Oliver and Gillian Austin for their support over many years, giving me the opportunity to pass these breathing techniques on to many more people than I would have been able to do alone.

My thanks are due to my willing models Lorraine Jeapes and Joan Coare, and my brother Robert Arcus. Finally, I must thank Alan, my husband, who read each chapter as it was written and rewritten and managed to keep me calm during the process.

Information for medical professionals

Many respiratory physicians and therapists now believe that a significant number of their COPD patients breathe in a dysfunctional way; and that this complicates their underlying respiratory disease. These patients need direction to correct their breathing, and this book has been written to help them to improve their day-to-day breathing.

Suitability of exercises

For the majority of people with COPD the breathing techniques in this book are completely safe to use. The exercises focus on calming breathing, awareness, nose-breathing and controlling coughing. The primary aims are to reduce hyperventilation, limit hyperinflation and increase fitness.

However, patients with severe and very severe COPD (including those who regularly use oxygen or those who have lost their normal respiratory drive) should approach the exercises with caution and only use what is helpful to them. The *knee bends* exercise (page 79) probably should be avoided by patients with severe COPD as it involves breath holding, which may not be helpful or pleasant for them.

Contraindications

It is recommended that the breathing exercises are not used by COPD patients who also have the following conditions:

- Severe emphysema with heart failure

- Kidney failure (especially if on dialysis)

- Current organ transplant (e.g. kidney, lung, liver, etc.)

- Previous brain haemorrhage or brain tumour

- Known arterial aneurysm

- Recent heart attack or stroke (three months)

- Lung cancer or any cancer requiring current treatment

- Active duodenal or stomach ulcer

- Uncontrolled high blood pressure

- Cardiac pacemaker device

- Sickle cell anaemia

- Schizophrenia

The medical conditions quoted here are for illustration only and do not represent an exclusive list.

1

Will breathing techniques help my COPD?

COPD stands for Chronic Obstructive Pulmonary Disease; it is an umbrella term used to describe a number of conditions, including chronic bronchitis, smoker's lung and emphysema. COPD leads to permanently damaged airways in the lungs, causing them to become narrower and making it harder to breathe.

When you have COPD your airways are not as healthy as they once were. But there is more to good breathing than just the width and condition of your airways – the *way* you breathe can make a real difference. For example, if you are climbing some stairs and deliberately breathe more quickly, perhaps thinking you'll get more oxygen in that way, you can inflate your lungs. Lungs that are full of air haven't got room to work properly and so, despite the extra effort, you'll still feel short of breath. In fact, your brain and body were giving you the wrong message – it's better to do the opposite and calm your breathing down.

During the next 28 days the aim is to replace the wrong messages such as 'Breathe more', with right messages such as 'Calm your breathing' so that your lungs work for you rather than against you. It does take time and a bit of willpower to overcome wrong automatic reactions, but once you have learnt to do so you will find your stamina increasing and your breathing will become much easier to control. The techniques can't repair damage to your lungs, but they can help you to breathe much more comfortably.

Make time for your health – it will pay dividends

In our society when we have a health problem there is a widespread belief that our doctor will be able to resolve it by providing medication, organizing surgery or arranging medical treatment. For many conditions this is true. Certainly there are medications available for COPD; but many people still continue to experience symptoms most days despite following standard medical advice.

The most effective way to treat COPD is through a joint effort involving your doctor, therapists, support from friends and family and most importantly yourself – you spending time working on improving your own health. Helping yourself is not as easy as taking a pill or going to the doctor, and it is a challenge to commit to regular exercises. You may not be used to dedicating much time to your own health; but consider this, that if you don't make time for your health then you are making time for illness. The vast majority of people who have already taken the time to follow this breathing exercise programme say that it is a price well worth paying; there are great benefits and some personal pride to be taken in managing your own condition.

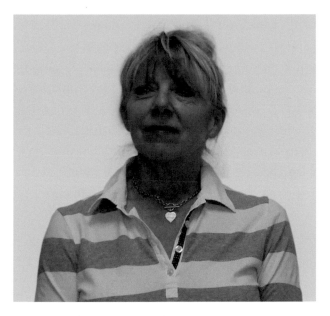

Nose-breathing is best!

Is there any evidence that these breathing techniques work?

There is evidence that breathing techniques do work – provided of course you take the time to learn them properly and practise them. Scientific trials have shown that people who have learned to breathe properly feel better and become more active. This in turn can reduce symptoms such as breathlessness and chest tightness.

There are lots of different breathing exercises in existence: childbirth exercises, breathing for army fitness training, meditation breathing, and more. This book describes therapeutic breathing techniques which are designed specifically to help COPD sufferers.

Are the techniques suitable for me?

Please check that your doctor is happy for you to give breathing techniques a try. The exercises in this book are primarily designed for people with mild to moderate COPD. Some of the exercises, such as those involving breath-holding, are not suitable for people with a severe condition or for those who are using oxygen on a regular basis. Also, if you have COPD and another medical condition, you must also check first with your doctor. In some conditions, such as diabetes and underactive thyroid, doing any form of exercise may change your need for medication.

What about my medication?

Continue to take your medication as prescribed. These are self-help techniques which are designed to be used alongside your usual medical care, in the same way as eating a good diet including plenty of fruit and vegetables. They are not an alternative treatment.

Smoking

If you are still smoking, then these techniques are unlikely to help you. The smoke you are inhaling will continue to irritate and damage your lungs. If you decide to stop smoking now and learn to breathe properly, you can give yourself the gift of a healthier, happier future.

2
What do I have to do?

Most people take breathing for granted and think about it only when it becomes a real issue, such as when they are hurrying to catch a train or climbing several flights of stairs. But people with a lung condition such as COPD, through necessity, are much more aware of their breathing on a minute-to-minute basis. Perhaps you hear yourself saying things such as:

- 'Breathing is hard work'
- 'I can't stop coughing'
- 'My chest feels tight'
- 'I get out of breath so easily'

Allow yourself a few minutes right now to try this taster exercise and hear yourself saying something different.

Rest back in a comfortable chair. Give yourself permission to relax for a few moments; you can't breathe properly if you are tense. Notice the movement of your chest as you take a couple of normal breaths in and out. Now just say the word 'Relax...' to yourself silently each time you breathe out. Continue for the next six breaths... Focus on breathing out... Close your eyes...

Better? Now let's get started.

How much time and effort?

For the next 28 days you need to put aside three 10-minute slots each day to practise the exercises and commit to a daily walk lasting around 15 minutes.

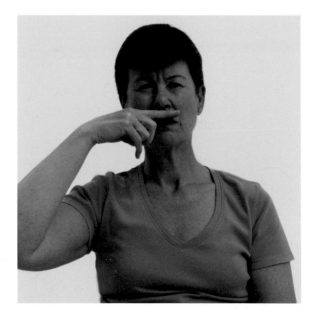

Feel your breath

Equipment

The only two pieces of equipment you need are an ordinary upright chair, such as a dining chair, and a watch or stopwatch to time yourself. Finding a stopwatch is much easier these days as most mobile phones have one built in.

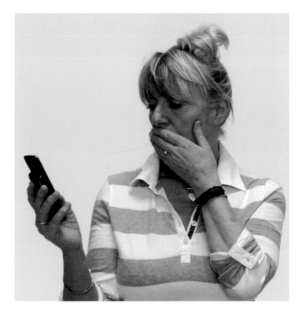

Time your breathing

Days 1–14: Basic skills

There are four essential skills that you will be learning:

- How to calm your breathing down

- A technique to reduce the frequency of coughing

- A walking exercise – to improve the way you breathe and your stamina

- An exercise to relax your breathing muscles

Days 15–28: Advanced skills

Once you have mastered the basic skills you should know what good breathing is, and be able to control some aspects of your breathing. Then you can move on to more active exercises which involve holding your breath and delaying your breathing for short periods of time.

Through these exercises you learn how to overcome breathlessness and feel more confident about controlling your condition. After 28 days you should be finding it much easier to calm your breathing down quickly when you feel short of breath.

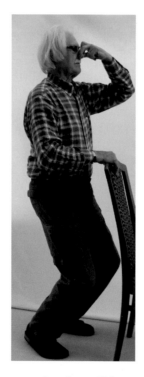

Overcoming breathlessness

Tips

Throughout the book there are tips on other aspects of life which can affect your COPD, such as how to avoid feeling short of breath on icy cold days and how to prevent laughing from turning into coughing.

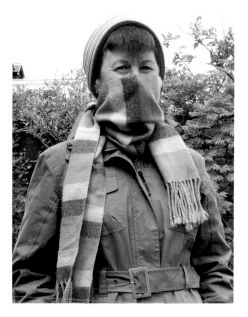

Breathe warm air on a cold day

Commit to the plan

If you do the exercises 'as and when' or 'more or less', then you are unlikely to feel much improvement. The 28-day plan appears simple, but actually it can be quite tiring. So follow the instructions, and fill in the chart on page 70 or 92 day by day. Don't overdo it! If you do experience problems, just stop, and start afresh the next day.

How do these techniques work?

Using breathing techniques in your daily life should help you to feel better in all aspects of your general health. Whether you are talking on the telephone or walking to the shops on a freezing cold day, you will start to automatically adopt a more comfortable way of breathing.

Breathing is an automatic, unconscious process – it just happens. This is a good thing because it means that you don't have to concentrate on controlling your breathing all the time and can get on with other things. However, like a lot of things you tend to do on automatic pilot (e.g. driving), it is easy to fall into bad habits after a while. This is what happens to many people with COPD. They feel breathless and their automatic reaction is to breathe faster, breathe heavier or cough. Unfortunately this usually makes things worse. By learning these breathing techniques you will start to lose the bad habits and adopt new, good breathing habits.

Where do the breathing techniques come from?

The practice of using breathing exercises to improve health goes back thousands of years. More than three thousand years ago the yogis in India were teaching yoga exercises called *pranayama* while the Chinese were employing similar techniques. These exercises are still used today by millions. Recently there has been a great deal of interest in new breathing techniques which were developed in Russia by Dr Buteyko. This 28-day plan uses an approach combining established breathing exercises, Buteyko and yoga exercises to help you to breathe freely and easily.

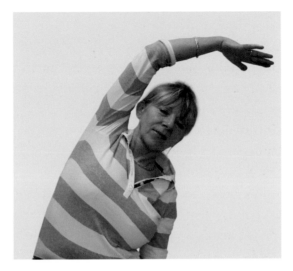

Stretch and breathe

Learning with a teacher

If you feel that you need to learn these techniques with a therapist, look for one who has specialist breathing exercise training. They can draw up an individual programme for you, focusing on what you would like to achieve. They will check that you are practising the techniques correctly and encourage you to keep to the programme. Contact your local COPD support group to locate a breathing teacher in your area (see page 94).

3
Feeling short of breath?

It can happen suddenly – one minute you are walking along chatting and laughing with friends, the next minute you are struggling for breath.

The *calm breathing* technique can provide you with a quick and easy option to help control your symptoms. The idea that you can overcome breathlessness simply by changing the way you breathe may seem ridiculous. Yet once you start to understand how you breathe, and how you can change your breathing, you can begin to see that this approach makes good sense.

What to do when you feel out of breath

We're going to jump in at the deep end and start with what to do when you feel out of breath. At this stage you don't know any of the breathing exercises in this book, so you need to follow the instructions step by step.

It's no good rushing around trying to find this book when you feel short of breath, so sit down in a comfortable chair and let's work slowly through the steps of the *calm breathing* technique now. When you come to use this exercise 'for real' it will probably only take a couple of minutes.

The calm breathing technique
1. Keep calm and rest forward

Whenever a slight feeling of breathlessness leads you to start breathing too heavily, then the first thing to do is not to panic but rather repeat to yourself 'Keep calm... Keep calm...'

This initial feeling of shortness of breath triggers an automatic fear response in your body, so the natural reaction is to feel agitated or anxious and to try to breathe as deeply as possible in as short a time as possible. If you have COPD, this is likely to make things worse.

Allow yourself to rest forward supported by a table (or garden wall or stair rail) or sit down. Lean forward but keep your back fairly straight. It may be helpful to loosen tight clothing, especially around your waist and neck. Move your knees apart so that your stomach can drop down.

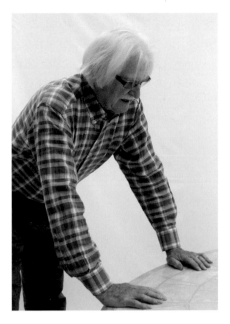

Keep calm and lean forward

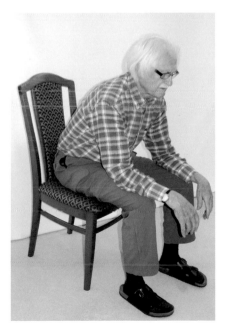

Let your stomach drop down

2. Change to nose-breathing

If you are breathing rapidly through your mouth, then try to change to nose-breathing. This is at the heart of many of the exercises. At first nose-breathing might be very difficult to control and you may need to do a mixture of nose-breathing *in* and mouth-breathing *out* for a short while. But as soon as you can, breathe only through your nose, both breathing in and breathing out. Your breathing might become noisier for a little while, but that's okay. (There's more on nose-breathing in Chapter 4.)

3. Reduce the flow of air

Put your index finger under your nose and feel the flow of the out breath on your finger. Now gradually, little by little, reduce the flow rate. Do this for at least six breaths. You might feel a really strong urge to gulp down lots of air, but resist and move on to the next step.

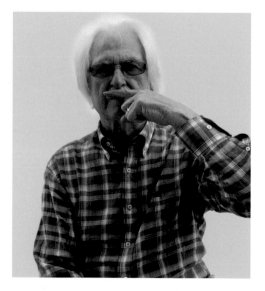

Reduce the flow of air

4. Slow down

Keep nose-breathing and keep your finger just under your nose. Now try to slow your breathing down by introducing a momentary pause after each breath out. This means after breathing out don't breathe in again for one second. Carry on doing this for at least six breaths. At first you might feel an urge to take a big breath, but resist and the feeling will quickly pass. There's more on this in Chapter 8.

5. Breathe less

Finally, if you are still breathing heavily, slightly reduce the amount of air you are breathing *in*.

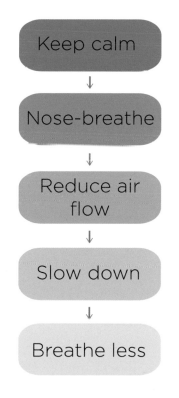

Calm breathing technique

By now you should be breathing easier and feeling better. If you are, say to yourself 'Well done! I controlled my breathing myself'; this will help to remind you to use *calm breathing* in the future.

Practise this sequence a few times so that you know exactly what to do when you next feel short of breath.

Tick the chart on page 70 each time you use this technique.

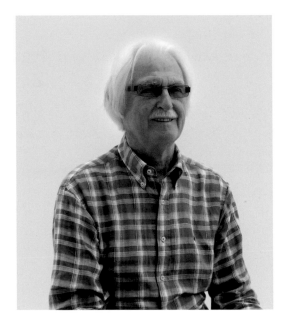

That's better

Why does this exercise improve my breathing?

When you feel short of breath, for any reason, your body moves into 'fight or flight' mode and your heart and breathing rate speed up because your body thinks you are in danger. You begin to breathe rapidly and heavily. Often there just isn't time for all the air that you breathe in to be breathed out. The lungs gradually inflate and air can become trapped; this triggers an even stronger feeling of breathlessness, making you want to breathe even more.

When you take control of your breathing, you can deliberately prevent yourself from breathing rapidly and heavily. By forcing yourself to adopt calm, gentle nose-breathing you give your lungs extra time to deflate and return to their normal size. As you become more confident, you will be able to do this quite quickly. Eventually you may be able to stop an attack of breathlessness before it starts.

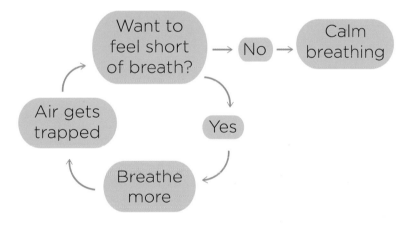

Control your breathing

Memory test

Can you remember the steps of *calm breathing* without looking back?

Write them here in your own words:

1. . . . .

   . . . .

2. . . . .

   . . . .

3. . . . .

   . . . .

4. . . . .

   . . . .

5. . . . .

   . . . .

Emma's story

Emma was 60 years old when she was admitted to a respiratory ward with a sudden worsening of her COPD. This was the first time she had been admitted to hospital since being diagnosed around eight years ago, and it was quite a shock. She stayed on the ward for seven days and was discharged feeling better, but quite anxious and unable to walk more than a few steps without feeling breathless.

Emma felt it was time to pay attention to her health. With the help of her doctor she started a

Stop Smoking programme, and with me she started breathing exercises.

Emma was slightly breathless all the time and the smallest exertion, for example, getting up to answer the door caused her to gasp for breath. Emma had been to a yoga class many years ago and was quickly able to relax; she realized that she was holding tension in her chest and shoulders and that when she relaxed, her breathing felt more comfortable.

We practised *calm breathing* several times sitting on the sofa. Then I asked her to imagine walking to the front door and back and then practising *calm breathing*. Then Emma did walk to the front door and back; she stopped herself gulping air and was able to get her breathing back to normal after a minute or so. For Emma's first week of practice I asked her to do three things:

1. To go through *calm breathing* once 'in her head', then to practise it 'for real', after walking to the door and back (or further if it was getting easier)

2. To breathe through her nose as much as possible

3. Just for the first week, to talk as little as possible

Emma's husband encouraged her to practise three times each day and soon she was walking to the village shop without feeling breathless. Three months on, Emma was delighted to tell me that she had stopped smoking and was feeling much better, both physically and mentally.

4
Breathing through your nose

Many people with COPD have a habit of breathing through their mouths, especially when they are exerting themselves in any way. The problem is that mouth-breathing irritates the lungs and reduces their efficiency.

Breathing through your nose while resting is often fairly easy, but more of a challenge is to overcome the urge to open your mouth when you are walking, going up stairs or being active around the house. Taking a *15-minute nose-breathing walk* every day will help you to master this. Walking is an excellent natural form of exercise; you may need to build up slowly if you haven't been very active for a while. If you are unsteady, or lacking in confidence, think about investing in a wheeled walker or 'rollator'; this may make you capable of longer excursions away from home and give you back your independence.

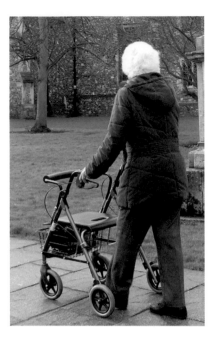

A rollator can give you back your freedom

A 15-minute nose-breathing walk

This 'breathing exercise' walk is different from a normal walk because you have to set yourself a little challenge – to breathe through your nose all the time. This means no talking – only walking! If you feel the need to open your mouth because you feel out of breath, then stop or slow down. Wait until you are able to continue walking with your mouth closed. You can always look in a shop window or at your watch if you feel self-conscious.

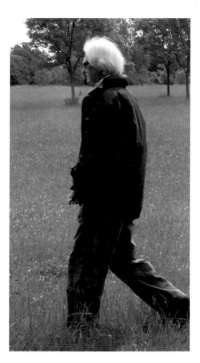

Walk, but don't talk

It can be very helpful to walk with a friend. Not only for encouragement and company, but also because they can do the talking if you meet anyone!

Tick the chart on page 70 or 92 each time you complete a walk.

Problems with walking

For some even a 15-minute walk will be too much in the beginning. Instead try just walking slowly around your home or go up and down a few stairs. The key points are to keep breathing through your nose and to calm your breathing so that it remains quiet.

It may be an idea during bad weather to take a walk around your nearest indoor shopping centre, where you can walk on the flat, in the warm, and enjoy a cup of coffee as a reward. If you are walking on a cold day though, make sure you cover both your nose and mouth. Cold air can irritate the lungs, even if you are breathing through your nose. Breathing through a scarf provides a warm air layer which helps to protect your lungs.

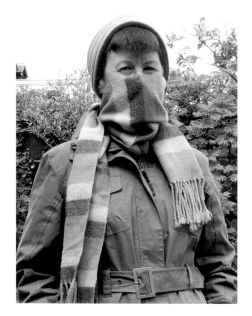

Cover your mouth and nose on an icy day

Your nose is a personal air-processing system

The nose is designed to be breathed through – it processes the air so that it is in a perfect condition for your sensitive lungs. The nose helps to protect the lungs by:

- Filtering out dust and pollen

- Moistening the air to keep your lungs healthy

- Warming the air to prevent cold air from irritating your airways

- Sterilizing the air to help kill off any bacteria and viruses

Breathing through your mouth does none of this, so it leaves your lungs vulnerable to damage and infection.

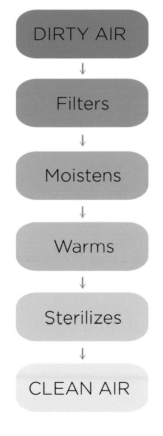

Nose-breathing

Breaking the mouth-breathing habit

Breathing through your mouth is understandable if your nose is permanently blocked. However, there are many people with COPD who don't have a blocked nose and yet still breathe through their mouth. What's more, they are often completely unaware that they are doing so. One clue to the fact that you may be mouth-breathing is if you often have a dry mouth. Another way to find out if you are an unconscious mouth-breather is to ask your family or friends whether they often see you with your mouth open.

Breaking the mouth-breathing habit is not easy. It may be something you have been doing for years without noticing. Therefore, in the early days you will probably need to give yourself frequent reminders. Useful strategies include:

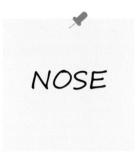

- Putting notes or small stickers around the house or at work. The stickers don't need to say anything, just as long as they remind you to nose-breathe.

- Setting a quiet alarm on your watch or mobile phone to remind you every hour through the day.

- Asking your family or friends to let you know when they see you with your mouth open. Often a simple, discreet, agreed sign is better than constantly hearing someone telling you to 'shut your mouth'.

It's impossible to breathe through my nose all the time!

When you are doing jobs around the house or need to get onto a bus quickly, it may be impossible to keep breathing through your nose. Instead, continue to breathe in through your nose, but breathe out through your mouth using a long, slow and controlled out breath. You may like to use this *pursed lips breathing* exercise:

Pursed lips breathing

1. Breathe in through your nose.

2. Purse your lips gently as if you were going to whistle.

3. Breathe out softly, taking your time. Breathe out twice as slowly as you breathed in. Let the air escape naturally; there is no need to force the air out of your lungs. Some people find it helps to make a soft 'sssssssssss' sound.

4. Return to breathing in and out through your nose as soon as it is possible.

Checking your nose

You may not feel you can breathe easily because your nose is blocked. To check – cover each nostril in turn and take three normal-sized breaths to check whether the other nostril is clear.

It is quite normal for one nostril to feel slightly clearer than the other but you should be able to breathe comfortably through either.

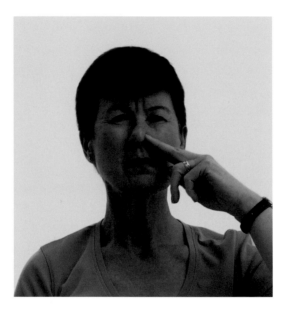

Check each nostril

If both nostrils are working well, that is very good news. If not, you will need to practise the following *nose-clearing* exercise.

Nose-clearing exercise
Repeat four times.
It can be helpful to read all the instructions before trying the exercise. Remember to keep your mouth closed throughout.

1. Pinch your nose
Sit down, take a normal breath in and a normal breath out. Then gently pinch your nose to prevent yourself from breathing in or out.

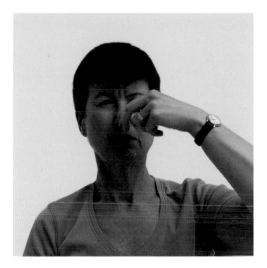

Hold your nose

2. Tip back and forward
Immediately tip your head backward and forward three times while holding your nose. Do this as quickly as is comfortable for you.

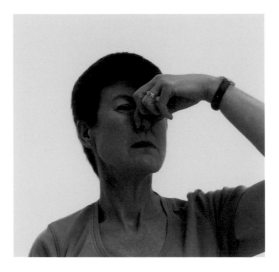

Tip your head back

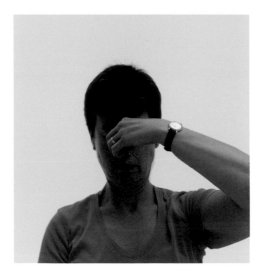

Tip your head forward

3. Breathe in gently

Keep your mouth closed and breathe in smoothly through both nostrils.

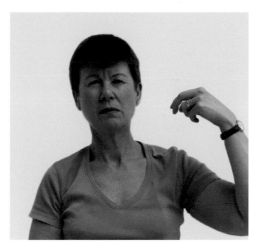

Breathe gently through your nose

4. Rest

Take a normal breath in and out through your nose.

Practise three times each day until you can breathe freely through both nostrils. This can take a week or two if you haven't breathed through your nose for many years.

Nose still blocked?

If you need to blow your nose, then do it very gently. Sometimes a salt-water nasal wash (available from a pharmacy) can help. If your nose remains very blocked, even after practising these exercises regularly for a couple of weeks, then consult your doctor for their advice.

Rachel's story

Rachel had asthma which used to be well controlled; but over the last two years she had been increasingly unwell and had been admitted to hospital three times. On the second admission the consultant told her she had COPD alongside her asthma and he gave her an additional inhaler to use. Rachel felt particularly breathless and wheezy when she moved between extremes of temperature, when she did even the slightest exercise, and when she was tired in the evening. Following the latest admission the doctor told her that he thought her breathing was 'dysfunctional' and suggested that breathing techniques might help her.

Rachel had problems with breathing through her nose; she constantly felt as if she were at the start of a cold. She had been allergy tested the previous year and was found to be allergic to dogs; unfortunately, she had four dogs at home.

It was likely that her dog allergy was part of the problem, but Rachel loved her dogs and could not consider living without them. I suggested she kept them out of the bedrooms, washed their bedding more frequently and regularly shampooed the dogs. Rachel was keen to feel better and quickly put all this into practice; she had a part-time job in the local cinema and did not want to lose her job through illness. Rachel struggled to fit the 28-day plan into her busy life, but she found the nose-clearing exercises worked well and she enjoyed the 15-minute walk, which often turned into a much longer walk with the dogs. At the end of the course Rachel said that changing to nose-breathing had been a 'revelation' for her and she felt it was the main reason that she was feeling so much better.

5
Controlling your cough

Is coughing always necessary? That may seem a strange question, but often people cough only because they have a tickle in their throat, not to clear phlegm. Imagine you are on holiday and visiting an old building. You go into a room; it is so dusty that it starts off a coughing fit, but why? As said earlier, the lungs are very sensitive to irritants such as dust, and this can make you want to cough. People who have normal lungs will probably cough as well, but they do not usually continue to cough.

In this dusty room, as you take a big breath in to cough, you breathe even more dust into your lungs. Not only that, the air you are breathing is cold, dry and fast-moving. So each time you take a big breath to cough, you inhale four cough triggers: dust, cold air, dry air and fast moving air. To stop this vicious circle you can use the *stop cough* technique.

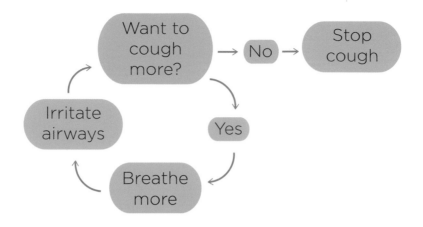

Try the *stop cough* technique

The stop cough technique

For this technique to work effectively, you need to use it as soon as you feel the first urge to cough. Practise with a 'pretend' cough to become familiar with the sequence. Do this several times, because if you are in a situation where you start to cough, everything will happen very quickly and you need to act equally quickly to stop the cough.

If you have a 'cough habit', you may need to use this technique very frequently at first, but as you become proficient at the technique your cough should settle down quite quickly. Overcoming the urge to cough is not easy and requires some willpower to maintain control. You may find it helpful to remember the *stop cough* as 'The four Ss' – Smother, Swallow, Stop and Smooth:

1. Smother the cough

As soon as you cough, or feel you are about to cough, put your hand over your mouth.

2. Swallow once

3. Stop breathing for two seconds

Take a small breath in and out through your nose. Hold your breath for two seconds (you don't need to pinch your nose).

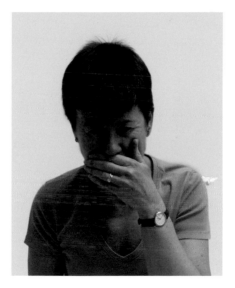

Smother, swallow and stop breathing for two seconds

4. Smooth breathing for 30 seconds

Breathe carefully and gently, keep your breathing smooth – as if you are trying to soothe your lungs. Continue for at least 30 seconds and keep your hand over your mouth.

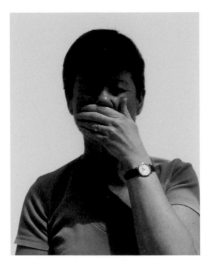

Breathe *smoothly* for 30 seconds

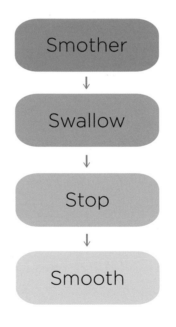

***Stop cough* technique**

Keeping your hand over your mouth increases your awareness of the urge to cough, making it easier to break the cough habit. Finally take your hand away from your mouth. If you still feel a tickle in your throat, repeat the technique from the beginning.

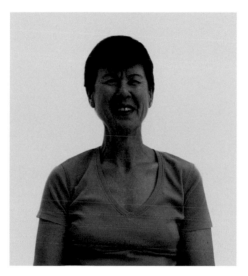

Repeat if necessary

Tick the chart on page 70 each time you complete this technique. It is hoped that you will find you are coughing less as the weeks progress.

Crunchy biscuits, eating and breathing

When people start to carefully observe what triggers a cough or shortness of breath, a common finding is foods with certain textures. Crunchy biscuits are a particular culprit; the small particles can be inhaled when you crunch, irritating the lungs and setting off a reaction. Notice what affects you; perhaps you need to eat fewer crunchy biscuits in future!

Some people with COPD feel an uncomfortable sensation in their chest after eating a large meal or need to stop to breathe during a meal. If this is the case with you, try very gently exhaling while you chew. It may take a bit of getting used to but can make a real difference to meal times.

Controlled coughing to clear phlegm

Often people with COPD have extra phlegm (mucus) in their lungs. As you practise nose-breathing and the *stop cough* technique, the amount of phlegm you make should decrease; but if you do need to bring up phlegm, you might like to try this short *controlled coughing* technique. When you practise this exercise, have the thought in your mind that you are allowed only one 'proper' cough to bring up the phlegm!

Follow these steps:

1. Use 'huffing' to move the phlegm to the larger upper airways

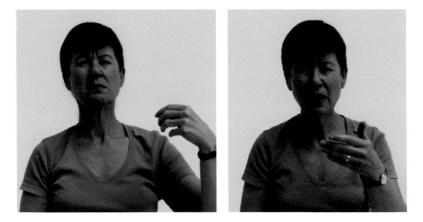

Breathe in – hold for 2–3 seconds – 'aaa...'

Sit comfortably with paper tissues to hand. Take in a normal breath through your nose and hold your breath for two to three seconds. Open your mouth wide and quickly lean forward as you breathe out, trying to force the air out of your lungs. Your breath should make a sighing, long 'aaaaaaaaah' sound.

Repeat this, but take a bigger breath in, and as you lean forward do a shorter, sharper breath out, making a shorter 'aaah' sound.

2. Not ready to cough up phlegm?

If the phlegm doesn't feel ready to come up, breathe gently for a couple of minutes, then repeat huffing once more. Avoid coughing if you can.

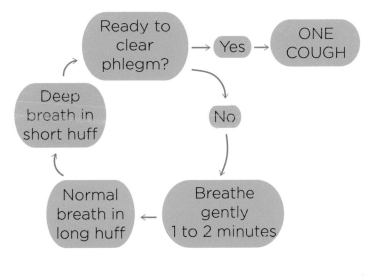

Controlled coughing technique

3. Ready to clear the phlegm?

Cough any phlegm into a paper tissue. One successful cough should do the trick. Briefly examine the colour of the phlegm (see 'Preventing chest infections' below) before throwing the tissue away.

4. Breathe gently to prevent more coughing

Breathe gently and use the *stop cough* technique to prevent you from coughing again.

If possible try to use *controlled coughing* no more than four times each day, as hard, persistent coughing can cause more harm than good and it is very tiring. You need some phlegm to help to protect airways from drying out, as well as acting as a trap for any dust or other particles that get into the lungs.

Large amounts of phlegm?

Most people who have completed this breathing plan have said that the amount of phlegm they produce is considerably reduced. But if phlegm is troubling you, then talk to your doctor and ask for a referral to a physiotherapist or physical therapist. They will be able to offer you several airway clearance options, such as a breathing device that uses vibration to help remove phlegm, postural drainage or a series of breathing exercises called the 'active cycle of breathing technique'.

Preventing chest infections

Wheezing, coughing and breathlessness can worsen if you have a chest infection. If you are coughing up yellow, green or blood-stained phlegm, then act quickly and visit your doctor for a checkup. Other signs to look out for are a high temperature, feeling disorientated or a sharp pain in your chest or shoulder.

Although chest infections aren't as contagious as colds and flu, they can be passed on through coughing and sneezing. So avoid close contact with people who are unwell. Washing your hands regularly can also help to prevent you from catching an infection.

Prevention is definitely better than cure! So it's a good idea to have the annual flu jab and the pneumonia jab.

If you have a chest infection

Follow your doctor's advice on medication and treatment. In addition you may find some of these tips helpful:

- Breathe through your nose as much as possible.

- Use a controlled coughing technique to clear phlegm.

- Rest in a fairly upright position; make yourself very comfortable, and use several cushions or pillows to support your back and head.

- Drink plenty of water or tea – these are better than fizzy drinks. Keep water with you and sip regularly. Your aim is to thin the phlegm in your lungs, making it easier to cough up.

- If your throat is sore, try a warm drink of honey and lemon.

Memory test

Can you remember the four Ss of the *stop cough* technique without looking back?

Write them here.

1. S ___ ___ ___ ___ ___ ___

2. S ___ ___ ___ ___ ___ ___

3. S ___ ___ ___

4. S ___ ___ ___ ___ ___

Deirdre's story

Deirdre had recently retired from her job as an office manager and was looking forward to spending more time on her hobbies. For the last year she had been suffering with an irritable cough, and six months ago was given a diagnosis of COPD. Her respiratory consultant suggested that she try breathing techniques to calm her cough. Deirdre said that sometimes she felt she couldn't get enough air in, but the main problem was 'the cough'.

'The cough' would often come on when she was cooking, cleaning the house, at the cinema or on the train, and once it started she couldn't stop it. Numerous times at the beginning of the session Deirdre would cough and clear her throat. We talked about the effect of coughing on her lungs and how a cough can become a habit, Deirdre quickly understood this and from that moment onwards used the *stop cough* technique.

Deirdre followed the plan with special attention to the *stop cough* and when she returned the following week she said she felt like a changed person. She was still working on nose-breathing, but she had found the *stop cough* technique completely effective. After another two weeks of practice Deirdre said that the breathing techniques had become a part of her daily lifestyle, her chest felt much easier and she just didn't cough any more.

6
Breathing more easily

Most of the time we don't think about our breathing – it just happens. However, to be able to control your breathing you need to become aware of how it changes from moment to moment; and you will learn this by assessing your own breathing. Once you are familiar with your own breathing pattern you can set about changing it for the better by learning the *relaxed breathing* exercise.

Remember that your breathing will not improve by just sitting and thinking about it. You must do the exercises to make it happen.

How are you breathing now?

Sit in an upright chair, place one hand on your lower chest and the other on your upper chest.

Let yourself relax for a moment and then answer the following questions.

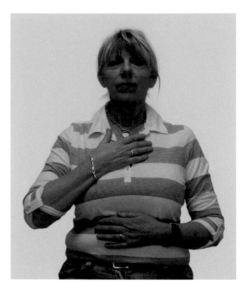

Put your hands on your chest

Q1. How fast are you breathing?

Use your watch to measure how
many breaths you take in one minute
(one breath is in and out).

_____

The ideal breathing rate is 12–16 breaths per minute.

Q2. Nose-breathing?

Are you breathing through
your nose?

Y/N

As you know, nose-breathing is healthier than
mouth-breathing.

Q3. Sighing or clearing your throat?

Is your breathing steady or is it
interrupted by...

Sighs
Sniffs
Coughs

Normal breathing is steady, smooth and gentle.

Q4. Where are you breathing?

Which hand is moving most? Or are
they both the same?

Upper
Lower
Same

Your lower hand should move most if you are
breathing properly.

Q5. How much movement is there in your chest?

Do you feel that your upper and
lower chest are both moving a lot?

Y/N

Sitting at rest, you should feel very little movement.

Q6. Quiet breathing?

Is your breathing noisy?

Y/N

Normal breathing is silent.

Q7. Are your chest muscles relaxed?

Do you feel any muscle tension in
your neck, back, shoulders, chest
or stomach?

Y/N

In an ideal world all your muscles would feel relaxed.

Now that you are aware of your breathing and know what correct breathing is, you can start to improve the way you breathe.

Relaxed breathing
1. Sit comfortably

Sit in a straight-back chair with your legs uncrossed. You may find a cushion behind your back makes this more comfortable. Make sure that the clothing around your waist is loose and not constricting your breathing.
Start the timer.

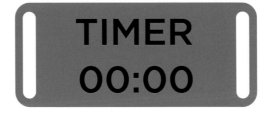

TIMER
00:00

2. Notice any tension?

Put your hands on your upper and lower chest and let yourself breathe smoothly and quietly through your nose. Perhaps ask someone to read these instructions to you – so that you can close your eyes.

Check your face, jaw, neck, shoulders, chest, stomach and legs for any tension and let yourself relax as much as you can. Keep breathing gently.

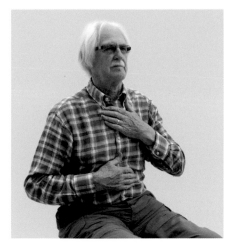

Check your body for tension

Next, focus on those areas of your body where you feel movement as you breathe.

After around a minute bring your top hand down to rest in your lap, if you wish.

3. 'Let go...' as you breathe out

Now concentrate on the area behind the hand on your lower chest. Feel a sense of 'letting go'. It can help if you say to yourself silently 'Let go' or 'Relax' each time you breathe out. You may find that your breaths become slightly smaller – which is good.

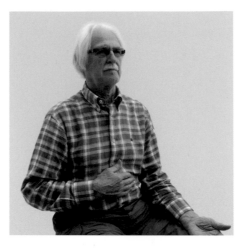

Breathe out and 'let go...'

4. Continue for three minutes, rest, then repeat once more

Practise *relaxed breathing* for three minutes.

Let yourself rest for around 30 seconds and then repeat the exercise once more.

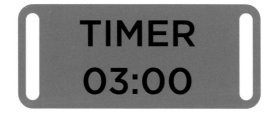

Try to practise *relaxed breathing* three times each day. It is easier to do this when your stomach is not full. Practising before breakfast can get the day off to a good start. You may want to complete a second practice before lunch, in the afternoon or early evening. Many people find that it is a good idea to do the final practice just before going to sleep as it also helps to relax the body.

Tick the chart on page 70 each time you complete a practice.

James's story

I first met James, age 75, after he had attended as an emergency at his local doctor's surgery, where the nurse had given him a nebulizer to ease his breathing. He felt better after being nebulized, but the nurse pointed out that he was still mouth-breathing and using his upper chest muscles to breathe. She suggested that a course of breathing techniques might help him. James was sceptical, but willing to give the techniques a try.

When he returned after two weeks of practice there was a definite improvement – he was now breathing properly. James was pleased; he said he had averted a panic attack by concentrating on his breathing and using *pursed lips breathing* until the feeling had passed. He was surprised that the techniques had made such a difference to his life. He found it easier to do the exercises lying on the bed with a couple of pillows behind his back. Now, he routinely did two rounds of *relaxed breathing* before his afternoon nap and at night before he went to sleep.

7
The Plan
Days 1 to 14

Finding the time to practise the breathing exercises regularly can be a struggle, so it pays to make sure you use the time you have as effectively as possible. Here are a few simple ideas on how to make the most of your practice sessions.

Choose the right place

Breathing exercises involve a good deal of concentration. Ideally you need somewhere quiet, with no distractions such as TV or music.

Make yourself comfortable

It is much easier to relax if the room is warm enough and you are wearing loose, comfortable clothes. Find an upright chair; put a small cushion behind your back if it makes you feel more comfortable. You should be able to place both feet on the floor. If your feet don't reach the floor, then put a cushion or book on the floor to rest them on.

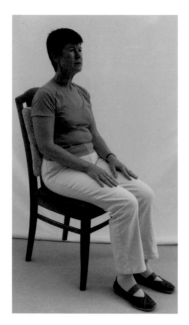

Are you sitting comfortably?

Keep everything you need in one place

It can be very frustrating if you have to hunt around for everything you need (e.g. book, pen, watch) when you want to practise.

Try to stick to a routine

Not only will this help you to practise regularly, but other people in your house will get to know when you need to be by yourself.

Think about what you want to achieve

Setting one or two realistic goals can help to keep you committed. For example, there may be things that you would like to do but would not consider doing at the moment because of your breathing problems. So, set modest targets to begin with. For instance, walking around the shops without becoming breathless or reducing how often you cough by a quarter.

Write your goals here

1. ....

   ....

   ....

2. ....

   ....

   ....

3. ....

   ....

   ....

Day 1–14 diary

Make a diary entry for each day that you do any practice. If you miss a day, or session, return to your breathing exercise routine as soon as possible.

Day 1–14 diary

Day	Daily walk	Calm breathing	Stop cough	Relaxed breathing	Notes
1 Monday	✓	✓✓	✓✓	✓✓✓	No coughing fits today, walk okay
1					
2					
3					
4					
5					

6				
7				
8				
9				
10				
11				
12				
13				
14				

Sue's story

Around four years ago Sue was walking to work, felt very unwell, and was admitted to hospital with a viral infection. After that, she experienced frequent chest infections and between these she suffered with a permanent dry cough. Sue felt shortness of breath when she carried out even small activities, such as hanging out the washing. Also, laughing and chatting always left her feeling extremely breathless. She said her life was quite miserable now. A friend of Sue's recommended she try breathing exercises.

Sue and her husband, Lee, both worked part time. It was New Year and they decided to work on the breathing plan together as their 'resolution'. Lee helped Sue to keep up a practice routine, recorded her results and walked with her. She needed to use the *stop cough* technique very frequently to stop her dry cough during the first couple of weeks. She also used a shortened version of the *stop cough* after laughing, to control her breathing. Gradually Sue felt more confident. She had a setback when she caught a cold but fortunately this time she didn't get a chest infection and she was able to resume the exercises after a week of rest.

After two months Sue and Lee were enjoying regular short walks. Sue still occasionally coughed and sometimes felt breathless, but Lee said that it was all much less troublesome than before. Sue said that she felt she had got her life back.

8
Reducing breathlessness

After two weeks of practice you should feel more confident about controlling your breathing. The focus now moves on to where you are breathing (it should be your lower chest) and how to build short breathing pauses into your *relaxed breathing* practice.

Understanding lower chest breathing

It is hoped that you are already breathing with your lower chest, but it is a good idea at this stage to check that you are doing this correctly.

The body's main breathing muscle is the diaphragm, located in the lower chest. It is a large flat muscle which is attached all the way around the inside of your lower ribs. If you breathe correctly, then your lower chest will move forward a little every time you breathe in, and as you breathe out it should relax back.

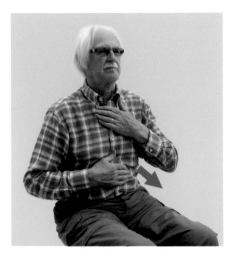

Breathe *in*: your *lower* hand should *move forward*

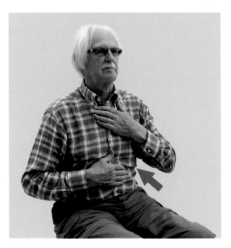

Breathe *out*: your *lower* hand should *relax back*

Lower chest breathing is the by far the most efficient way to breathe, and, if you breathe this way all the time, it can improve your energy levels. People with COPD often use the muscles in their upper chest, shoulders and neck to help them to breathe, but this style of breathing is inefficient and very tiring. If you relax the muscles around your shoulders and upper chest at every opportunity, after a few days your breathing should begin to change to a natural, easier, lower chest breathing pattern.

It is worth noting that you won't gain any benefit by actively pushing your lower chest forward or pulling it back, because this will increase the amount of tension in your muscles. So just be patient.

Becoming less sensitive to breathlessness

Feeling short of breath automatically puts the body on a 'fear alert', often without you being aware that it has happened. The trouble with fear is that it is a strong stimulus to increase your breathing – completely the opposite from what you are trying to achieve with the exercises. This is why calming and controlling your breathing is such an important part of managing your symptoms.

One method that people use to control fear is called 'systematic desensitization' – that is, to become gradually less sensitive to it. This is the approach used here; by repeatedly exposing yourself to mild shortness of breath, you gradually learn to reduce your fear response.

Fear can build upon fear, and some people with COPD find that they begin to feel less confident and so avoid doing some of the things they used to enjoy. For example, fear of being embarrassed about having to take medication in front of a group of people, or the fear of having a coughing fit, or even being afraid of upsetting family arrangements through being unwell. The ability to 'fine tune' your breathing can help you to overcome these fears.

Breathing with pauses

1. Settle yourself

You are already familiar with *relaxed breathing* so the next step is to become comfortable with one-second pauses between breaths.

As before, sit comfortably in a straight-back chair with your legs uncrossed. Put your hands on your upper and lower chest and settle yourself by breathing smoothly and quietly through your nose.

Quickly check your face, jaw, neck, shoulders, chest, stomach and legs for any tension and let yourself relax as much as you can. Then place your top hand on your lap.

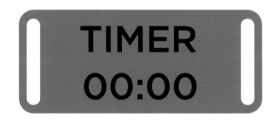

2. Pause between breaths

Now begin to pause momentarily after each breath out...and just before the next breath in. In other words, delay breathing, but in a totally relaxed way, as if you are waiting for the next breath in.

You might start to experience a slight shortness of breath; try to relax when you feel this sensation. If the sensation becomes too strong, return to *relaxed breathing* or take a couple of larger breaths.

You can rest your other hand on your lap if it helps to relax your shoulders.

Continue practising for three minutes.

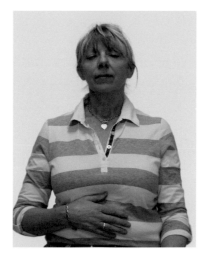

Wait for the next breath

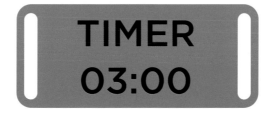

TIMER
03:00

3. Repeat once more
Allow yourself to rest for around 30 seconds and then repeat this three-minute exercise.

Tick the chart on page 92 each time you complete a practice.

Hardly breathing at all?
This exercise replaces *relaxed breathing* in your daily routine. Practise regularly and you will find that you will be able to pause your breathing for longer than one second. Allow this

to happen but don't force it. After several days of practice you may find that you feel as if you are hardly breathing at all, which is excellent news. It shows that you have gained really good control of your breathing.

Talking and laughing

You have probably noticed that it's hard to keep breathing through your nose when you are talking or laughing. But carry on talking and laughing! Just be aware that talking, laughing, shouting, sighing and crying can also cause you to mouth-breathe and to breathe too heavily. While your friends continue to talk or laugh, you can practise *breathing with pauses* to counteract this. Try it, no one will notice that you are doing anything unusual! This can often prevent your breathing getting out of control in social situations and will boost your self-confidence.

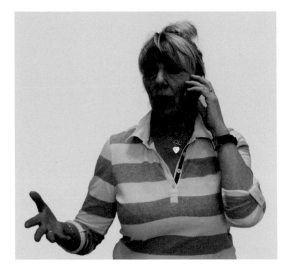

Are you talking too much?

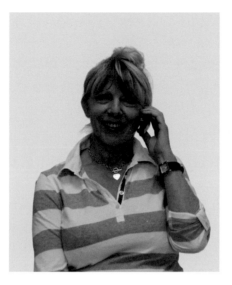

You may want to listen more!

Knee bends

Let's move on to an active exercise which may be quite challenging at first. The key to success, as with all these techniques, is to 'give it a go', but also to know when to stop.

If you have severe COPD, this exercise may not be suitable for you. Please check with your doctor.

Only breathe through your nose, and keep your breathing slow. Do this exercise once each day in place of one of your *relaxed breathing* slots.

1. Take hold of a chair

With one hand, hold onto a chair or table to help you to balance.

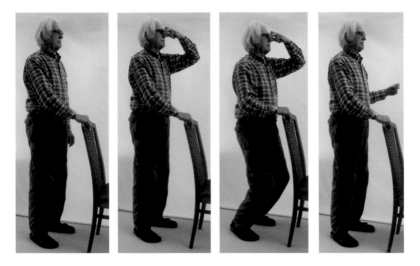

**After breathing out – pinch your nose – bob
up and down – breathe in *gently***

2. Pinch your nose

Breathe in *and out* gently, then with your other hand lightly pinch your nose to hold your breath.

3. Bob up and down 2–10 times

Keep holding your breath as you bend your knees, and then straighten them until you feel a *little* short of breath. Initially try two knee bends to get the hang of it.

4. Release and breathe gently through your nose

Release your nose and breathe in *gently*. If you need to take a big breath in or need to open your mouth, then you have done too many knee bends. Start again with fewer knee bends.

Record the number of knee bends on the chart on page 92.

Over the next 14 days, gradually increase the number of knee bends, until you are able to do ten and can still breathe easily when you release your nose.

Duncan's story

Duncan said to me, 'I want to enjoy my retirement without constantly focusing on my breathing'. Duncan had an active life, travelling extensively with his wife to Caravan Club events. His breathing problem had started suddenly – one morning he woke up on holiday feeling unable to breathe. He was given a diagnosis of mild COPD and two inhalers, one of which was a reliever inhaler that he used several times each day.

Duncan was very organized; he had been a naval engineer for many years. He drew up a computerized timetable to make sure he practised all the exercises exactly as requested and made notes of any questions and problems that arose.

He found *relaxed breathing* challenging initially. He noticed that he was breathing with his upper chest and holding his stomach tight. To overcome this he wanted to force his lower chest to move, but realized he must try to relax instead. It took over a week before he could 'let go' enough to allow his lower chest to move naturally. He said it was a great feeling and reminded him of times in his naval past when he was coming home on leave.

Duncan stuck with the breathing techniques, and his shortness of breath and chest pain became less frequent. He continued with the exercises after the 28 days as he felt he was still improving. Three months later and he rarely used his reliever inhaler. Duncan reckoned that most of his improvement was as a result of learning to breathe properly with his lower chest. An excellent result he felt, and well worth the effort.

9
Stretching for better breathing

Now it's time to use your new breathing-control skills alongside physical movements to improve your posture and mobilize your spine and chest. These exercises follow a more structured approach, aiming to integrate breathing into movement, which should also help you to breathe better when going about your daily activities.

Hold up the sky
Repeat five times.
You can do this exercise standing or sitting.

1. Breathe in as you lift your arms
Breathe in while you lift your arms up slowly, as if you are lifting your hands up towards the sun.

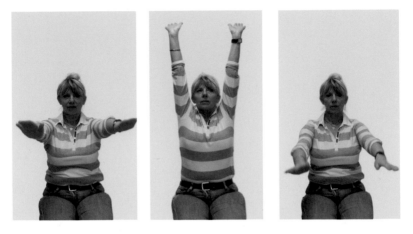

Breathe in – hold – breathe out slowly

2. Hold your breath, tip your hands back

Now hold your breath for a couple of seconds (yes, this time you are holding your breath after breathing in!) whilst moving your hands and fingers back – as if you are holding up the sky.

3. Breathe out as you lower your arms

Lower your arms slowly. Try to synchronize your breathing with the movement.

Don't breathe out too far; just breathe out to the point where you would normally breathe in again. At first you might like to take a gentle breath between each movement, but as you progress you might be able to do all five repetitions in succession.

Elbow circles
Make five circles on each side.

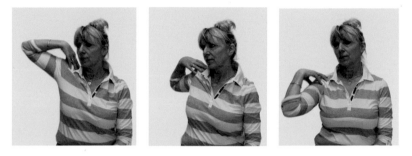

Lift your shoulder – elbow back – draw a circle

1. Place your hand on your shoulder and rotate your elbow

Place your hand lightly on your shoulder and slowly rotate your elbow in a circle, first up, then back, then down and back to where you started. Co-ordinate your breathing with the movement; breathe in as you lift your shoulder and elbow, and breathe out as you lower your elbow and bring it forward.

2. Repeat on the other side

Gentle twist

Repeat three times on each side.

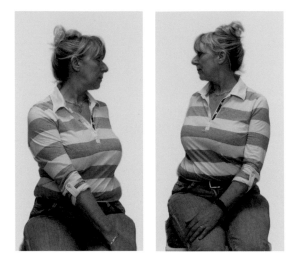

**Straighten up, then twist – turn your
head gently to look behind you**

1. Straighten up, put your hand on your opposite knee and twist gently

Straighten up your spine. Put your right hand on your left knee, twist gently and slowly to the left while breathing out. Don't strain. Take hold of the back of the stool or chair with your left hand and turn your head gently to the left to look behind you. Stay there for 5–10 seconds, breathing very gentle, small breaths. Return to face forward with a slow breath in.

Rest for 10 seconds.

2. Twist to the right

Sideways bend
Repeat three times on each side.

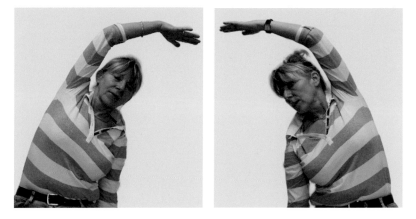

Stretch up, then bend

1. Breathe in as you stretch your right arm up, breathe out as you bend to the left

Breathe in as you stretch your right arm up towards the ceiling; keep that feeling of stretch as you take your arm over to the left. Notice the stretch in the side of your waist and chest. Stay there for 5–10 seconds, breathing very gentle small breaths. Come back to the starting position.

2. Lift your left arm, stretch up and bend to the right

Remember to tick the chart on page 92 after your stretching session.

Diana's story

Diana had lived with COPD for over 15 years. She was a member of her local COPD support group and regularly attended her local chest clinic. She had followed a pulmonary rehabilitation programme, which she had found helpful; she had good control of her breathing and kept herself as active as possible. She wondered if these new breathing techniques could add anything to what she was doing already.

Diana noticed that she often took large mouth breaths, especially when she was active. When she started nose-breathing while walking, she was amazed to find that she felt less tired than usual.

Diana found holding her breath during the *knee bends* challenging, but she noticed that her tolerance of breathlessness was building up, and she was determined to do ten knee bends without opening her mouth. She first succeeded in doing this on Day 26!

The stretching exercises were a particular favourite. Diana said she would continue to do these, and the *knee bends*, every day as they only took a few minutes. She was keen to recommend new exercises to her friends at the support group and her respiratory nurse.

10
The Plan
Days 15 to 28
and beyond

Aches and pains?

Physical chores, such as cleaning the windows or gardening, can leave you aching the next day. We recognize that this is a short-term ache and it's often an indication that you may have overdone it.

The *breathing with pauses*, *knee bends* and *stretching* exercises can similarly cause temporary side effects, such as aches or mild headaches, especially if you have done very little exercise over a long period of time. If you do experience side effects, then first try increasing your fluid intake. If you are still achy, cut down your breathing exercise practice to once or twice each day instead of three times. You may need to continue to practise the breathing exercises for more than 28 days to achieve your goals, but gradually you will get there.

Why do I feel short of breath?

The feeling of being short of breath develops when you breathe less than your body thinks you should at any particular time. Everyone has experienced this feeling at some point in their lives, even if it was only on the school sports field, and it can feel very unpleasant.

At first the idea of deliberately creating shortness of breath may seem alarming or unnatural; after all, we are often advised to trust that our body knows best. However, this is not always the case. Take the situation with an insect bite. There is an overwhelming desire to scratch and scratch again, yet doing so only makes things worse; it's best to resist the urge to scratch. Likewise, if you are feeling short of breath, there is an overwhelming desire to breathe in more air and still more air; yet doing so only makes things worse. It's best to resist the urge to breathe more.

Day 15–28 diary

Make a diary entry for each day that you do any practice. If you miss a day, or session, try to return to your breathing exercise routine as soon as possible.

Completed the 28-day plan?

The goal of practising breathing techniques is to help you get the most out of every breath, enabling you to live life to the fullest with COPD. By the time you reach this stage, if you wish, you can stop practising *relaxed breathing* or *breathing with pauses* on a daily basis. To maintain your fitness you may want to continue with the *stretching* exercises and the *15-minute nose-breathing walk* and build these into your daily routine.

There may be times in the future when your breathing comes under stress due to particular events or ill-health and you will want to return to using the exercises. However, this usually does not need to continue for very long.

Getting more active

Perhaps you are 'on a roll' after the 28 days! Once you are confident with controlling your breathing during the *stretching* exercises, it may be time to embark upon a new activity to tone up your muscles. We're not talking treadmills or gyms here! Consider joining a gentle fitness class, walking group, yoga class, short mat bowls or whatever appeals to you. Alternatively, you might prefer an exercise DVD or sport simulation computer programme that you can use at home. There is a really good reason for you to do this. If you haven't exercised for a while your muscles may take time to become 'toned up'. But, if you can improve your muscle fitness by keeping up your daily walk and doing some gentle exercise every week, it is likely that your stamina will increase. This regular exercise should also make you feel healthier and you can integrate breathing exercises such as *nose-breathing* and *breathing with pauses* into the sessions for maximum benefit.

Day 15–28 diary

Day	Daily walk	Breathing with pauses	Knee bends	Stretching exercises	Notes
15 Friday	✓	✓✓✓	4/5/5	✓	Shoulders feel stiff. Enjoyed walk
16					
17					
18					
19					
20					

21						
22						
23						
24						
25						
26						
27						
28						

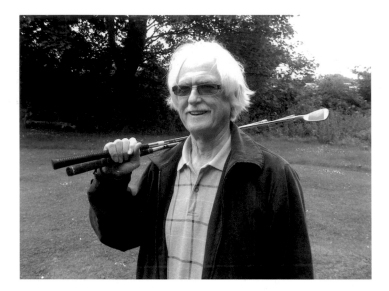

Getting more active!

Pulmonary rehabilitation

Ask your doctor about pulmonary rehabilitation courses at your local hospital or clinic, as these are a recommended treatment for COPD. It's worthwhile taking up the opportunity to attend one if you can.

Support groups

Having an illness like COPD can feel quite isolating. Most people find it very helpful and reassuring to use the services of support groups; many of these are charities which can provide specialist care at home and in community clinics. You can get all the up-to-date information you need to make informed decisions and enjoy a better quality of life.

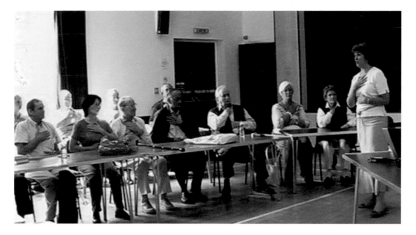

A COPD support group trying some breathing techniques

The support groups encourage people to chat, exchange ideas and get together. No one understands how it feels to live with COPD better than other people with COPD. You can share your experiences through groups or internet web forums if you prefer. There are local support groups throughout the world and contact details can be accessed through the internet or ask your doctor or nurse.

Please spread the word!

Congratulations on reaching the end of the book. If you have found the exercises beneficial, then please tell other people. The pharmaceutical industry has a multimillion-pound advertising budget to tell doctors and nurses about new drugs, but there is no advertising budget to tell them about COPD breathing exercises! It is up to you to tell your friends, your doctors and your physiotherapists that the techniques have helped you, even if just a little. Then more people will have the opportunity to try these simple, yet powerful techniques designed to help you live well and breathe well.

Jack's story

Jack had suffered with mild asthma when he played football at school, but he hadn't experienced any breathing problems since his teens. He had a physically hard job working as an animal farmer. During the last year he started to notice that he was 'struggling to catch a breath' and was feeling chest pain, especially when working in cold weather and walking uphill. His doctor sent him for heart and lung tests. His heart was fine, but he was told he had COPD and was given some medication. Three months on, despite using the medication, Jack was still feeling breathless and said he was willing 'to do what it takes' to manage his breathing better, so he started the 28-day breathing plan.

Before he began, it was clear that Jack's breathing was fast and noisy and that he was breathing mainly through his mouth. After the first week of following the plan, Jack reported that it had been a struggle to change to nose-breathing; when he was working, his automatic reaction was to change to a fast, mouth-breathing pattern. He said that if he made himself breathe through his nose, he felt very breathless for a few seconds, but the feeling quickly passed. He could then carry on, although he needed to slow down a little.

It took Jack another three weeks to master all the exercises. After four weeks he was feeling 'almost back to normal' with no breathlessness or chest pain, and he also said that he was sleeping better.